BODY BUILDING DIET FOR WOMEN

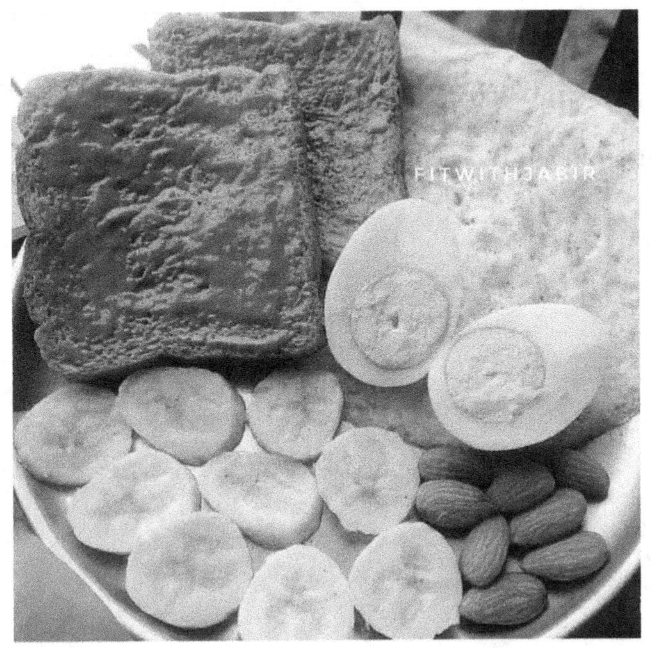

Comprehensive step by step guide to bodybuilding, healthy eating and meal plans, with pre workout nutrition strategy

EPIPHANY HUB PRINTS

BODY BUILDING DIET FOR WOMEN

COPYRIGHT © [2024] BY [EPIPHANY HUB PRINTS]

TABLE OF CONTENT

INTRODUCTION

Welcome to the ultimate resource for women-only bodybuilding dietary advice. You've found the ideal website if you're looking for an in-depth analysis that covers the fundamentals of efficient nutrition for strength and muscle gain as well as the particular issues and difficulties faced by female bodybuilders.

The number of women participating in bodybuilding and fitness has increased dramatically in recent years. More than ever, women are embracing the liberating adventure of body-sculpting, defying preconceptions, and putting their all into reaching their fitness objectives. But even with all of the knowledge out there, it can be difficult to sort through the complexities of nutrition specifically designed for female bodybuilders.

This book is meant to be your reliable travel companion, offering you a road map to help you negotiate the subtleties of nutrition unique to female bodybuilders. This book is for people of all skill levels, whether you're a novice hitting the gym for the first time or an experienced athlete trying to improve your technique.

Why This Particular Book?

This book is not your average reference to bodybuilding diets. It transcends one-size-fits-all strategies and formulaic meal regimens. Rather, it provides an in-depth exploration of the science underlying nutrition, equipping you with the knowledge and comprehension necessary to make decisions that are in line with your individual objectives and body type.

This book's comprehensive approach to women's bodybuilding nutrition is what makes it unique. We are aware that following strict diet regimens or monitoring macros won't get you the body you want. It's about putting your general health and wellbeing first, feeding your exercises, and maximizing your performance.

What to Anticipate:

You will go on a voyage of discovery in the pages that follow as you learn the foundational principles of nutrition designed especially for female bodybuilders. Every chapter has been painstakingly designed to give you useful insights and doable tactics, ranging from knowing your calorie and macronutrient requirements to planning your meals for optimal performance.

We'll explore the science of supplements to fill in any nutritional shortages, the significance of adequate hydration, and the function of micronutrients in supporting your body's operations. You'll discover how to pay attention to your body's signals, modify your diet plan in light of your objectives and advancements, and get past typical obstacles encountered by female bodybuilders.

But theory is not the only topic of this book. It has to do with real-world application. Along with meal planning advice and techniques to help you make nutrition a seamless and pleasurable part of your lifestyle, you'll find a plethora of delectable and nourishing recipes designed to assist your bodybuilding journey.

In the end, this book serves as more than a manual. It is a friend, an instructor, and a reliable ally in your pursuit of realizing your greatest potential as a female bodybuilder. Therefore, this book is here to help you every step of the way, whether your goal is to achieve a stage-worthy physique, smash personal records in the gym, or you just want to feel strong, confident, and empowered in your own skin.

Are you prepared to start this life-changing adventure? Now let's explore and discover the best dietary strategies for female bodybuilders.

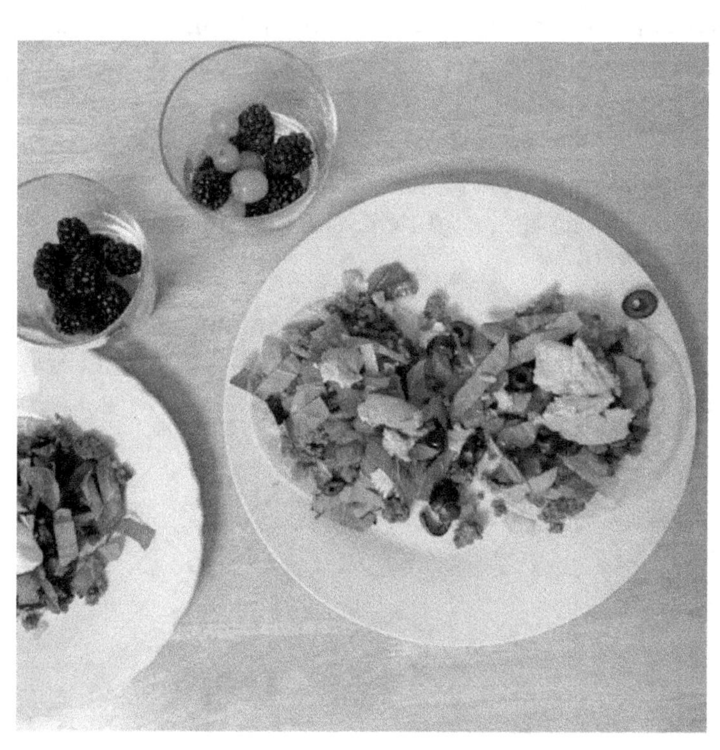

CHAPTER ONE

INTRODUCTION TO WOMEN'S BODYBUILDING NUTRITION

Understanding the Unique Nutritional Needs

Women's bodybuilding showcases the strength and tenacity of the female physique via a dynamic blend of athleticism, strength, and aesthetics. But beneath the sculpted muscles and spectacular lifts, there is a complicated interaction of physiological elements that determines the nutritional needs specific to women bodybuilders.

Women's unique hormonal changes and metabolic complexities require a customized approach to diet, unlike that of men. Hormonal fluctuations can have a substantial impact on energy levels, food utilization, and muscle protein synthesis during menstruation and menopause. This can affect bodybuilding performance and recuperation.

Furthermore, compared to men, women usually have a higher percentage of essential body fat, which is necessary for vital physiological processes including hormone synthesis and reproductive health. Dietary planning requires precision since it provides a sophisticated challenge to balance the requirements for hormonal health with the demand for leanness.

Importance of Nutrition in Achieving Fitness Goals

Nutrition becomes a key component of success while aiming for fitness goals because it has an unrivaled effect on body composition, performance, and general well-being. Nutrition becomes more than just food for women involved in bodybuilding; it becomes a tactical weapon for maximizing athletic potential, encouraging muscle growth, and speeding up recupcration.

Using the proper ratio of protein, carbs, and fats to fuel exercise creates the foundation for improved strength, endurance, and metabolic efficiency. In particular, protein plays a critical function in boosting muscle synthesis and repair, which in turn promotes hypertrophy and makes it easier to recover from strenuous training sessions.

Moreover, carbohydrates replenish glycogen stores and support performance during strenuous workouts, acting as the main energy source for high-intensity activity. It is critical to balance the consumption of carbohydrates with each person's unique energy needs and training demands in order to maximize athletic performance and maintain metabolic health.

In the meanwhile, dietary fats are important for women who bodybuild because they support satiety, cellular integrity, and hormone production. Women can sustain hormone balance, improve the absorption of fat-soluble vitamins that are crucial for general health, and promote cognitive function by include healthy fats from foods like avocados, almonds, and olive oil.

In addition to macronutrients, clever calorie management and nutrient scheduling become crucial tactics for reaching fitness objectives in women's bodybuilding. Women can maximize their athletic potential by coordinating nutrition and training cycles in order to maximize metabolic responses, promote muscular growth, and enhance recovery.

Essentially, nutrition is the cornerstone that helps women bodybuilders achieve athletic excellence by enabling them to shape their bodies, maximize their performance, and develop a long-term attitude to health and wellness. In the fast-paced world of bodybuilding, women can break through barriers, surpass constraints, and redefine what it means to be an athlete by utilizing the power of customized nutrition.

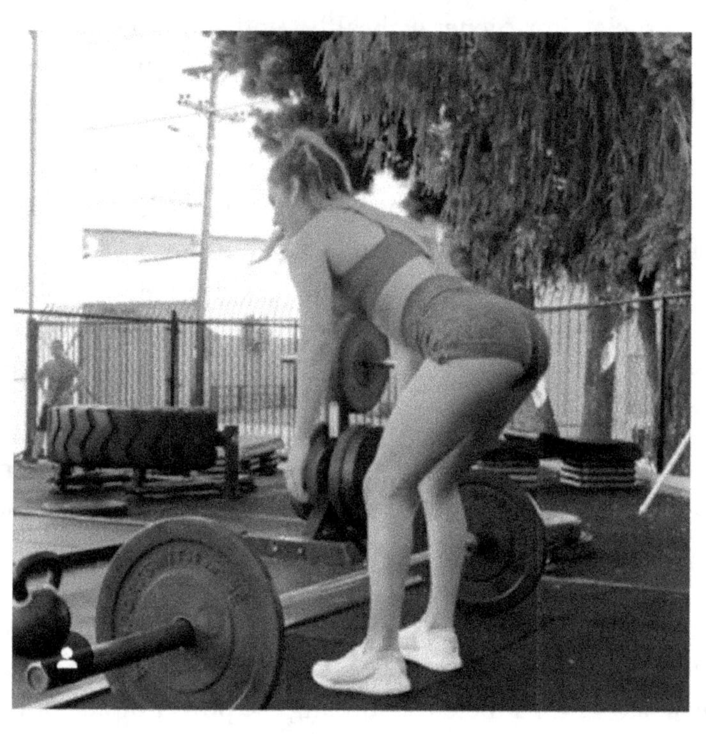

CHAPTER TWO

ESSENTIAL MACRONUTRIENTS FOR WOMEN

Lean muscle mass growth, repair, and maintenance in women are significantly aided by protein, which is frequently heralded as the foundation of muscle building. Knowing the subtleties of protein requirements in the context of women's bodybuilding diet is crucial to maximizing results, improving recuperation, and reaching fitness objectives.

Protein's Role in Muscle Building

Since it contains the amino acids required for both muscle growth and repair, protein is the main component of muscle tissue.

A sufficient protein intake is essential for developing muscle hypertrophy and strength increases during resistance training and bodybuilding.

Assessing Protein Requirements:

The amount of protein needed varies depending on age, body type, degree of activity, and fitness objectives.

In order to assist muscle repair and recovery, women who regularly engage in resistance training or severe physical activity may have increased protein needs.

How to Determine Your Protein Intake:

For inactive people, general recommendations indicate a daily protein intake of 0.8 to 1.2 grams per kilogram of body weight.

Depending on training intensity and goals, women who actively participate in bodybuilding or strength training may benefit from consuming more protein, 1.2 to 2.2 grams per kilogram of body weight per day.

Sources of Superior-Grade Protein:

A comprehensive amino acid profile, which is necessary for muscle protein synthesis, is ensured by including a range of protein sources.

Fish, poultry, turkey, lean beef cuts, and lean meats like chicken are all great sources of high-quality protein.

Proteins derived from plants, such as lentils, quinoa, tofu, and tempeh, supply the essential amino acids needed to create muscle.

Timing and Distribution of Protein Intake:

Evenly distributing your daily protein intake promotes optimal recovery and long-term muscle protein synthesis.

Before and after resistance training sessions, eating meals or snacks high in protein can improve muscle repair and recovery.

Additional Points to Consider:

Although the primary source of protein should be whole foods, there are easy ways to meet higher protein needs, particularly after exercise, with protein supplements such whey protein, casein, or plant-based protein powders.

Utilizing Protein and Staying Hydrated:

Sufficient hydration is necessary for muscle growth and the best possible use of proteins. Water is essential for the movement of nutrients, the creation of proteins, and the elimination of waste from muscle cells.

Achieving optimal muscle growth, improved recovery, and peak performance in women's bodybuilding nutrition requires an understanding of the significance of protein and the ability to customize intake to match specific needs. Women can reach their maximum potential in bodybuilding and strength training by emphasizing foods high in protein and carefully balancing their diet with supplements.

Importance of Healthy Fats in a Balanced Diet

Understanding the significance of macronutrients is crucial for women's bodybuilding nutrition in order to achieve optimal performance, muscle growth, and general well-being. The three macronutrients that make up a balanced diet are protein, carbs, and fats. Each is essential for providing the body with energy and supporting a range of physiological processes.

Protein

Because it is essential for muscle growth, repair, and maintenance, protein is frequently referred to as the foundation of women's bodybuilding nutrition. Adequate protein intake is critical for maximizing muscle protein synthesis and improving post-exercise recovery for women who participate in regular strength training or bodybuilding exercises.

Furthermore, eating foods high in protein helps increase satiety, which supports overall metabolic health and helps with weight management.

Sources: seitan, tofu, tempeh, poultry, fish, eggs, dairy products, legumes, and plant-based protein powders.

Recommended Intake: Depending on personal objectives and activity levels, aim for a daily protein intake of 1.2 to 2.2 grams per kilogram of body weight.

Carbohydrates:

The body uses carbohydrates as its main fuel source, especially during periods of high-intensity exercise and severe training. Carbs are essential for bodybuilders because they help women restore their glycogen stores, maintain energy levels, and perform at their best throughout exercises. Carbs are also necessary for facilitating muscle glycogen resynthesis, accelerating recovery, and reducing exhaustion after exercise.

Sources: minimally processed carbohydrate sources, fruits, vegetables, legumes, and starchy vegetables (such as sweet potatoes and squash).

Recommended Intake: Prioritize complex carbs and sources high in nutrients, and consume carbohydrates based on your own energy requirements and activity level.

Healthy Fats:

Healthy fats are an essential part of a balanced diet for female bodybuilders, even though they are sometimes disregarded. Healthy fats are not just a concentrated source of energy; they are also essential for cellular function, hormone production, and nutrient absorption. Including a range of healthful fats in your diet can help maintain joint health, hormone balance, and general wellbeing.

Sources: fatty fish (such as salmon, mackerel, and sardines), flaxseeds, chia seeds, hemp seeds, avocado, nuts, seeds, olive oil, and coconut oil.

Recommended Intake: To maintain overall caloric balance and nutrient needs, aim to include a range of healthy fats in your diet while reducing portion sizes.

Women's bodybuilding diet must include a balanced intake of major macronutrients, including as protein, carbs, and healthy fats, to support muscle growth, optimize performance, and enhance general health and vitality. You may properly feed your body, improve athletic performance, and fulfill your bodybuilding dreams by giving priority to nutrient-dense meals and customizing your diet to fit individual goals and energy demands.

CHAPTER THREE
MICRONUTRIENTS AND WOMEN'S HEALTH

Role of Vitamins in Supporting Fitness

Vitamins in particular are essential for maintaining women's health and fitness, especially when bodybuilding is involved. Women who participate in intense training and bodybuilding activities have a greater need for micronutrients to support a variety of physiological processes that are critical to their overall health, recuperation, and performance. It's critical to comprehend the unique functions of vitamins in connection to female bodybuilding in order to maximize training results and reach peak fitness.

Vitamins are organic substances that the body needs for a variety of biochemical processes, such as immune system response, energy metabolism, and muscle repair. In the world of women's bodybuilding, a number of vital vitamins are essential for maintaining fitness objectives.

Vitamin D: Also known as the "sunshine vitamin," vitamin D is necessary for strong bones, a healthy immune system, and healthy muscles. For women bodybuilders, adequate vitamin D levels are essential because they promote calcium absorption, bone mineralization, and muscle function, all of which lower the risk of fractures and improve overall athletic performance.

Vitamin C: Due to its potent antioxidant properties, vitamin C is essential for shielding cells from oxidative stress brought on by strenuous exercise. Additionally, it promotes the synthesis of collagen, which is necessary for the upkeep of healthy connective tissues like tendons and ligaments. This lowers the danger of injuries that are frequently sustained during weightlifting and bodybuilding exercises.

Vitamin E: Vitamin E is another powerful antioxidant that guards against the harm that free radicals, which are produced during vigorous exercise, can do to cell membranes. Furthermore, vitamin E may facilitate speedier healing and muscle repair by mitigating oxidative stress and inflammation brought on by exercise.

Vitamin A: Beneficial for skin health, eyesight, and immunity, vitamin A also promotes general well-being in female bodybuilders. It contributes to immune system and skin integrity maintenance, which is important for promoting recovery from hard exercise and avoiding infections that could impede training advancement.

B vitamins: The B-complex vitamins, which include cobalamin (B12), thiamine (B1), riboflavin (B2), niacin (B3), pyridoxine (B6), folate (B9), and thiamine (B1), are essential for the synthesis of red blood cells, energy metabolism, and neurological function. These vitamins are necessary for the body to convert proteins, fats, and carbs into energy, which enhances performance and endurance during demanding exercise sessions.

Vitamin K: For women who lift weights and participate in resistance training, vitamin K is essential for blood coagulation and bone health. It also helps to maintain strong bones and avoid fractures.

Vitamin B12: Beneficial for nerve function and energy metabolism, vitamin B12 helps women bodybuilders maintain their power and stamina.

Apart from these vital vitamins, other micronutrients like minerals and antioxidants are also crucial for promoting women's health and fitness in the bodybuilding setting. It is imperative that women bodybuilders incorporate a diversified, balanced diet high in foods that are high in micronutrients, as well as tailored supplementation as needed, to ensure adequate vitamin consumption and support their overall health and fitness goals.

Minerals and Their Impact on Performance

There are other factors outside macronutrients like protein, carbs, and fats that contribute to peak performance and muscle building. Essential minerals and other micronutrients are critical for hormone balance, general health, and sports performance. In the bodybuilding environment, knowing how minerals affect women's health is critical to optimizing gains, improving recovery, and fostering long-term wellbeing.

Calcium

Significance for bone density and health, which is essential for preventing osteoporosis, a condition that affects many women, particularly as they age.

supports nerve transmission, muscular contractions, and general muscle function—all of which are necessary for bodybuilding performance and strength.

Iron:

essential for maintaining energy metabolism, minimizing weariness and low energy, which are common problems for active women, and transferring oxygen in the blood.

Due to reduced oxygen delivery to muscles, iron deficiency can hinder performance, recuperation, and muscle growth. This might result in diminished strength and endurance.

Magnesium

contributes to the synthesis of proteins, energy production, and muscular function—all of which are vital for the growth and repair of muscles.

enhances cardiovascular health, nervous system modulation, and bone health, all of which are related to general performance and wellbeing.

Zinc

Important for protein synthesis, wound healing, and immune system function; particularly important during periods of rigorous exercise; also essential for recuperation and immune system maintenance.

supports the synthesis of testosterone, which is essential for women's muscle growth and strength, as well as hormone balance.

Potassium and Sodium:

Electrolytes are essential for nerve transmission, muscular contractions, and fluid balance, particularly in hot conditions and during vigorous exercise.

Sustaining electrolyte balance is crucial for avoiding cramping in the muscles, staying hydrated, and promoting optimal performance and recuperation.

Selenium

functions as an antioxidant, aiding in muscle repair and recovery by shielding cells from oxidative stress and inflammation brought on by rigorous exercise.

enhances immune system health, metabolism, and thyroid function, all of which are factors in overall health and performance.

Phosphorus:

vital for the synthesis of energy, bone health, and muscle function; supports bodybuilding performance and recuperation overall.

contributes to the creation of ATP, the main cellular energy currency that powers muscular contractions during exercise.

In the context of bodybuilding, it is critical to comprehend the function of these vital minerals and their effects on women's health in order to maximize performance, enhance muscle growth, and promote general well-being.

The benefits of these micronutrients for female bodybuilders can be maximized by incorporating a balanced diet rich in nutrient-dense foods and thinking about possible supplementation under the supervision of a medical expert or certified dietitian.

CHAPTER FOUR

CALORIC INTAKE AND ENERGY BALANCE

For women who build their body, gaining muscle mass is a complex process that necessitates a thorough comprehension of energy balance and calorie consumption. This part explores the complexities of calculating calorie requirements that are specifically designed for women to gain muscle, offering a thorough road map for maximizing your nutrition strategy and properly fueling your body for growth and performance.

Understanding Basal Metabolic Rate (BMR) and Total Daily Energy Expenditure (TDEE):

The concept of Basal Metabolic Rate (BMR), or the amount of calories your body requires to maintain basic physiological activities at rest, is the cornerstone of calorie intake and energy balance. Your BMR is influenced by various factors, including age, height, weight, and body composition.

Your BMR is included in Total Daily Energy Expenditure (TDEE), which also includes the calories you burn from physical activity and the thermic effect of meals. Your daily calorie needs can be more precisely estimated by calculating your TDEE, which takes into account your lifestyle and degree of exercise.

Calculating the Calorie Requirement for Muscle Gain:

Consuming a caloric surplus—consuming more calories than one expels—is crucial for bodybuilding muscle gain. To minimize fat gain and maximize muscle growth, the amount of this excess should be carefully calculated.

For women to gain lean muscle mass, a moderate caloric excess of about 250–500 calories above your TDEE is often advised. This excess reduces the chance of gaining too much fat while supplying the energy needed to support muscle growth.

Monitoring Intake of Macronutrients:

The distribution of macronutrients—protein, carbs, and fats—along with calorie consumption, is critical for promoting muscle growth and overall bodybuilding performance in women.

Consuming protein is especially important for the growth and repair of muscles. Aim for 0.8–1 grams of protein per pound of body weight per day to assist the synthesis and repair of muscle proteins.

The body uses carbohydrates as its main energy source, especially during vigorous exercise. To fuel your exercises and replace your glycogen levels, include complex carbs in your diet, such as those found in whole grains, fruits, and vegetables.

Good fats are necessary for the synthesis of hormones, the health of joints, and general wellbeing. To enhance peak performance and recovery, include foods high in healthy fats, such as avocados, nuts, seeds, and fatty fish, in your diet.

Monitoring Progress and Adjusting Caloric Intake:

To make sure that your calorie intake is in line with your muscle building objectives, it is imperative that you regularly assess your progress. Monitor your overall performance, strength increases, and changes in body composition to determine how well your nutrition strategy is working.

Based on your personal training response and results, modify your calorie intake as necessary. To maintain a moderate surplus and maximize muscle building while avoiding fat buildup, gradually raise or decrease your calorie intake.

Women's bodybuilding calorie requirements for muscle gain must be calculated strategically, balancing energy intake and expenditure. Understanding the fundamentals of energy balance and calorie intake, recording your consumption of macronutrients, and keeping an eye on your progress can help you customize your diet plan to promote lean muscle gain and successfully meet your bodybuilding objectives.

Balancing Energy Intake and Expenditure in Women's Bodybuilding

Women's bodybuilding success demands not just commitment to training but also careful consideration of diet and nutrition. Understanding the delicate balance between calorie intake and energy expenditure is essential to this. We will go into the nuances of energy balance and calorie intake in relation to women's bodybuilding in this extensive book, giving you the information and tactics you need to maximize your performance and reach your fitness objectives.

Comprehending Caloric Intake:

The quantity of calories obtained from food and drinks is referred to as caloric intake. When it comes to bodybuilding for women, calorie consumption is essential for supplying the energy required for training, muscle growth, and general metabolic processes. But there are other equally significant aspects to take into account, such as the amount and type of calories consumed.

Finding Your Calorie Requirements:

One of the most important steps in bodybuilding nutrition optimization is determining your calorie demands. Your calorie requirements are influenced by a number of factors, including your activity level, muscle mass, basal metabolic rate (BMR), and your goals (such as fat reduction or muscle building). Knowing these things, utilizing reliable calculators, or consulting a licensed nutritionist can assist you in figuring out your individual calorie requirements.

Balancing energy intake and expenditure: When the number of calories consumed and the number of calories expended are equal, energy balance is reached. For women bodybuilders to achieve particular fitness objectives, such as maintaining weight, decreasing fat, or gaining muscle, energy intake and expenditure must be balanced. While taking fewer calories than expended leads to fat loss, a positive energy balance (consuming more calories than expended) encourages muscle building.

Strategies for Balancing Energy Intake:

It takes careful consideration of both the quantity and quality of calories consumed to achieve a balanced energy intake. Pay attention to nutrient-dense foods that supply important macronutrients (carbohydrates and protein).

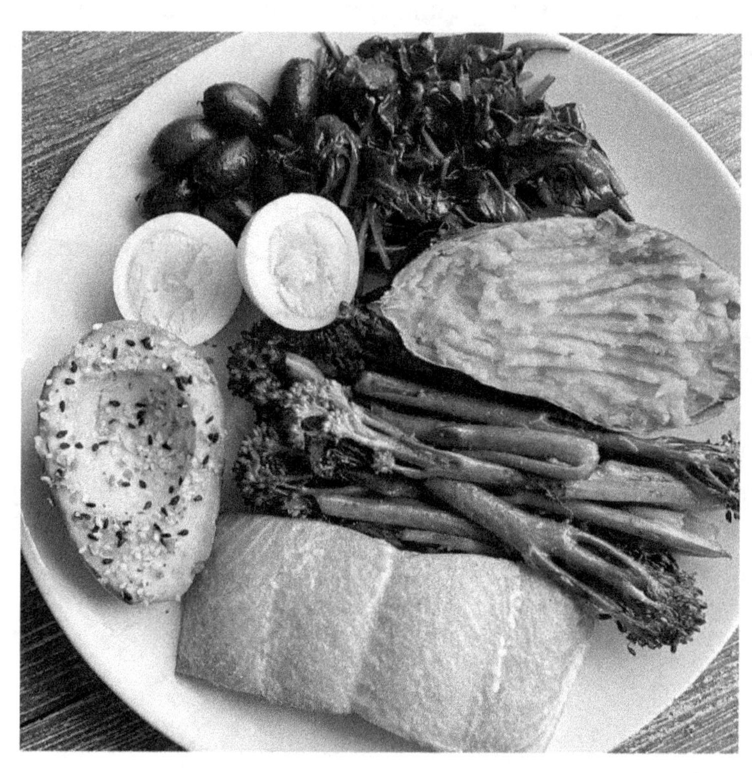

CHAPTER FIVE

STRATEGIC MEAL PLANNING FOR MUSCLE BUILDING

Pre-Workout Nutrition Tips

Any bodybuilding routine must include pre-workout nutrition since it supplies the fuel required to enhance performance, endurance, and muscle growth. Optimizing pre-workout diet can help women specifically gain strength, assist their recovery, and maintain high energy levels during training sessions. In this extensive book, we explore the nuances of pre-workout nutrition designed with female bodybuilders in mind, providing helpful advice and techniques to maximize the effectiveness of your sessions.

The Time Is Crucial: Try to eat a well-balanced lunch or snack around one to two hours prior to working out that includes carbohydrates, protein, and healthy fats. This guarantees that nutrients are easily accessible to power your workout session by providing enough time for digestion and absorption.

Protein for Muscle Growth and Repair: To promote muscle growth and repair, prioritize your protein consumption prior to working out. Choose high-quality sources including fish, chicken, eggs, dairy products, lean meats, and plant-based substitutes like tofu, tempeh, lentils, and grains high in protein.

Carbohydrates for Energy: During intense exercise, carbohydrates are the main fuel source since they replenish glycogen stores and give you long-lasting energy. To properly fuel your workout sessions, choose complex carbs like those found in whole grains, fruits, veggies, and starchy vegetables.

Healthy Fats for Sustained Energy: To promote hormone production and offer sustained energy, include healthy fats in your pre-workout meal or snack. You can incorporate avocado, nuts, seeds, and nut butter into your pre-workout nutrition plan as these are great sources of healthy fats.

Hydration Is Essential: Especially during strenuous exercise, proper hydration is essential for both performance and recuperation. To maintain optimal fluid balance and avoid dehydration, make sure you are adequately hydrated before exercising by consuming water or electrolyte-rich beverages.

Steer Clear of Heavy or High-Fat Meals: Although it's crucial to incorporate healthy fats into your diet before working out, steer clear of meals that are too heavy or high-fat as they could cause pain when working out. For a more digestible option, go with lighter options to avoid stomach problems when working out.

Take into Account Individual Preferences and Tolerance: Try out a variety of pre-workout meal selections

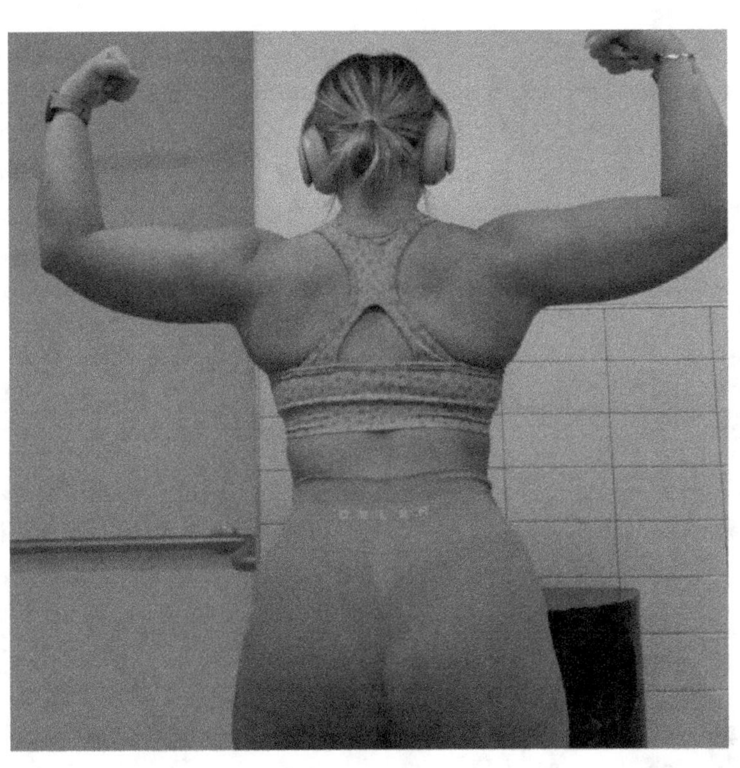

to find what suits your body and tastes the best. Depending on their energy demands and tolerance, some women might prefer a modest snack, while others would choose a larger lunch.

Supplementation: To improve performance and endurance, if necessary, think about combining pre-workout supplements like caffeine, beta-alanine, or branched-chain amino acids (BCAAs). However, before incorporating any supplements into your routine, speak with a medical expert or qualified nutritionist.

Pay Attention to Your Body: Observe your body's reaction to various pre-workout meals and snacks. To maximize your workouts, modify your nutrition plan according to your energy levels, performance, and general well-being.

Consistency Is Key: Last but not least, to optimize performance gains and foster long-term advancement in your bodybuilding journey, give consistency top priority in your pre-workout dietary regimen. Maintaining a regular eating schedule and supplying your body with the nutrition it needs to perform at its best throughout training will guarantee that your body gets the nourishment it needs to flourish.

You can effectively attain your fitness goals as a female bodybuilder and maximize your performance by incorporating these pre-workout dietary advice into your plan. Prioritize well-balanced meals, sufficient water, and personal preferences to energize your exercises and reach your maximum potential in the gym.

Post-Workout Nutrition Strategies

Any woman's bodybuilding path must include post-workout nutrition because it is essential for muscle growth, recuperation, and overall performance improvement. You can maximize your progress in gaining lean muscle mass by carefully scheduling your meals to enhance recovery, refill glycogen stores, and repair damaged muscle tissue after hard training sessions.

We'll explore the essential elements of post-workout nutrition plans designed especially for female bodybuilders in this extensive article.

The Timing is Crucial: The optimal time for your post-workout meal is crucial for promoting muscle growth and recovery. Try to have a well-balanced lunch with carbs and protein within 30 to 60 minutes of finishing your workout. This window, which is also known as the "anabolic window," occurs when your body is most responsive to the absorption of nutrients, promoting the growth and repair of muscles.

Protein for Muscle Repair: For female bodybuilders, protein is essential to their post-workout diet. Eating lean meats, chicken, fish, eggs, dairy products, or plant-based foods like lentils or tofu helps provide your muscles with the critical amino acids they require for growth and repair. To maximize muscle protein synthesis after a workout, aim for a high-protein supper that has 20–30 grams of protein.

Carbohydrates for Glycogen Replacement: Carbohydrates, in addition to protein, are essential for restoring the glycogen stores that are lost during vigorous activity. Choose complex carbohydrates that have a low to moderate glycemic index, including those found in whole grains, sweet potatoes, fruits, and vegetables, to help muscle recovery and offer a gradual release of energy without quickly raising blood sugar levels.

Healthy Fats for Satiety and Nutrient Absorption: You may improve the absorption of fat-soluble vitamins and antioxidants as well as encourage satiety by including a little amount of healthy fats in your post-workout meal. To promote general health and wellbeing, include unsaturated fat sources in your post-workout meals, such as avocados, nuts, seeds, and olive oil.

Drinking water for Recovery: Since dehydration can hinder muscle growth and performance, water is an essential part of diet after exercise. Make sure you stay properly hydrated by sipping water before, during, and after your workout. If you engage in lengthy or severe activity, you should think about drinking an electrolyte-enhanced water or sports drink to replace the electrolytes you lose via perspiration.

Nutrient-Dense Whole Foods: Make sure your post-workout meals include nutrient-dense whole foods to provide your body the vitamins, minerals, and antioxidants it needs for healing and general well-being. For a balanced and fulfilling post-workout meal, choose a range of vibrant fruits and veggies, lean proteins, whole grains, and healthy fats.

Customized Nutrition Strategy: Keep in mind that different people may have different post-workout nutritional requirements based on things like training volume, intensity, and personal objectives. To properly support your bodybuilding journey and satisfy your specific nutritional needs, pay attention to your body's signals of hunger and satiety and modify your post-workout meals accordingly.

Meal Examples and dishes: We've compiled a list of sample meals and dishes that are specifically designed for female bodybuilders to assist you in incorporating these post-workout nutrition methods into your meal planning. These meals will highlight scrumptious and nutrient-dense options that help with muscle recovery, enhance performance, and accelerate your quest for your fitness objectives.

Carefully considering post-workout nutrition techniques designed especially for female bodybuilders is an important part of strategic meal planning for muscle gain. Protein, carbs, healthy fats, hydration, nutrient-dense whole foods, and customized nutrition strategies are essential for maximizing muscle recovery, boosting performance, and reaching your bodybuilding objectives.

Watch this space for recipes and sample meals that will help you improve your nutrition after a workout and gain more lean muscle mass.

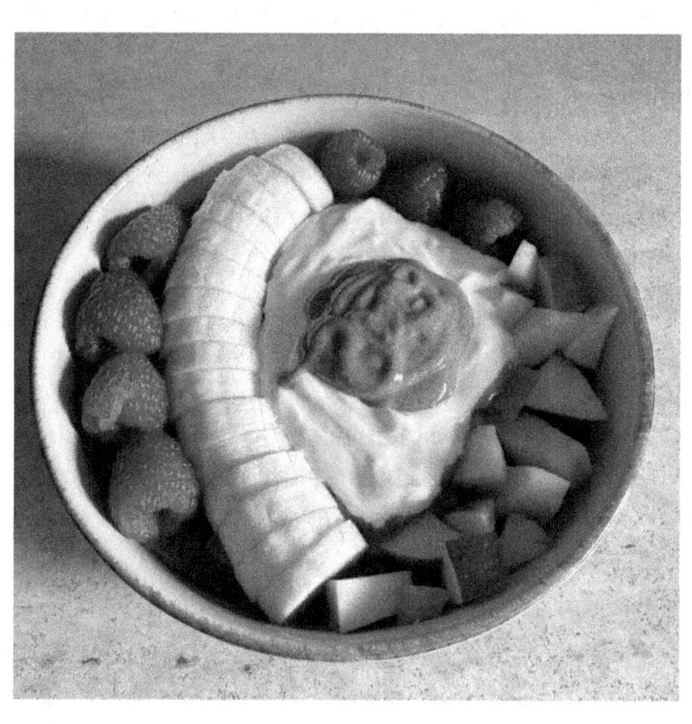

Timing Meals for Optimal Results

You may support general health and vigor while building and maintaining lean muscle mass by intelligently timing your meals throughout the day. We explore the nuances of meal scheduling for female bodybuilders in this extensive article, offering helpful tips and methods to help you get the most out of your efforts.

Understanding the Timing of Nutrients:

Macronutrient Timing: Timing your intake of fats, proteins, and carbs to coincide with your exercise sessions in order to promote energy production, glycogen resupply, and muscle repair.

Meal Frequency: Investigating the advantages of having regular, well-balanced meals that are evenly spread out throughout the day to promote satiety, muscular protein synthesis, and metabolism.

Strategies for Nutrition Before Exercise:

Timing: When to eat before working out to maximize energy, improve performance, and reduce tiredness during workouts.

Macronutrient Composition: Eat meals low in fat to aid in digestion, moderate in protein to help muscle repair, and high in carbohydrates for energy that is available quickly before working exercise.

During Exercise Fueling:

Importance of Intra-Workout Nutrition: Understanding the role that electrolytes and carbohydrates play in sustaining energy levels, hydration, and performance over extended training sessions highlights the significance of intra-workout nutrition.

Strategies for Hydration: adding electrolytes and fluids to maximize performance and avoid dehydration during strenuous exercise.

Nutrition for Post-Workout Recovery:

Anabolic Window: Examining the idea of the anabolic window following exercise and how it affects the timing of nutrients and muscle repair.

Protein Timing: To promote muscle regeneration, glycogen replenishment, and recovery, it's critical to have a balanced post-workout meal or snack high in protein and carbohydrates.

Nutrition Before Bed:

Nighttime Recovery: Techniques for maximizing the growth and recuperation of muscles during the night, such as bedtime snacks or supplements high in casein and slow-digesting protein.

Tailored Strategies for Timing Meals:

Organizing Mealtimes to Fit Your Schedule: modifying meal timing plans to take into account personal preferences, exercise regimens, and timetables.

Pay Attention to Your Body: observing signs of hunger, energy levels, and performance to modify the timing and makeup of meals as necessary.

Long-Term Food Scheduling:

The Secret Is Consistency: highlighting how crucial it is to eat at regular times and consume the right nutrients in order to maintain healthy eating, performance, and muscular growth.

Meal Prep & Planning: Strategies for efficient meal preparation and scheduling that guarantee access to wholesome meals and snacks all day long.

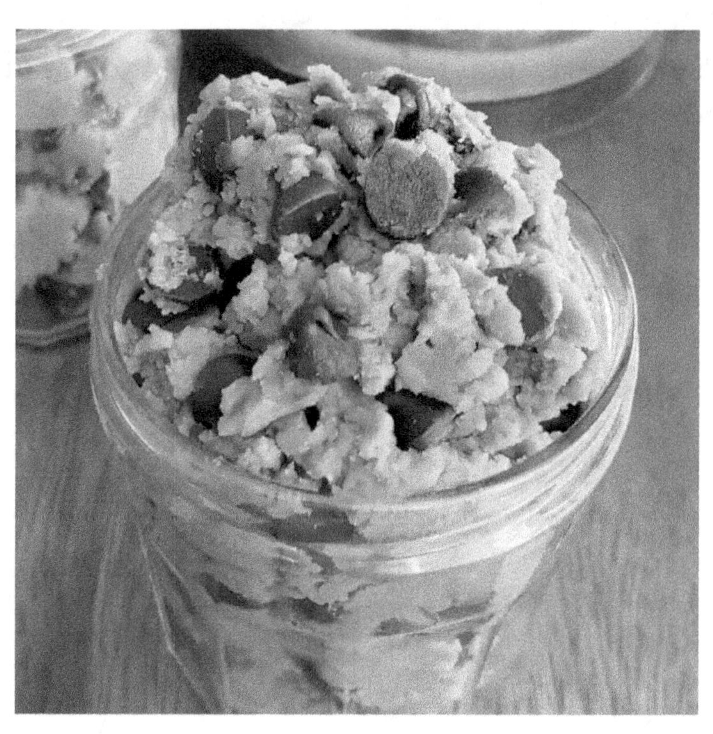

CHAPTER SIX

HYDRATION FOR WOMEN IN BODYBUILDING

Importance of Water for Performance

In order to achieve peak performance and general health, especially in the context of women's bodybuilding, hydration is essential. In addition to being necessary for living, water is also a basic component of many physiological processes, including as waste elimination, temperature regulation, and nutrition transfer. Adequate hydration is critical for bodybuilders to maximize muscular function, support recovery, and maximize athletic performance.

Because of the extra strain that severe resistance training and muscle-building activities put on the body, it is especially important for women to maintain optimal hydration levels. Dehydration can affect muscular recovery, reduce strength and endurance, and degrade physical performance, all of which can reduce the efficacy of training programs.

For this reason, it is imperative that ladies who aspire to be successful in the bodybuilding industry comprehend the significance of water and put tactics in place to guarantee proper hydration.

The immediate impact that adequate hydration has on muscle function and performance is among the main advantages it offers women bodybuilders. Since water makes up around 75% of skeletal muscle, even mild dehydration can result in notable reductions in muscle strength and power output.

Sufficient hydration prioritises proper muscular contraction and coordination during resistance training sessions, enabling women to lift larger weights, complete more repetitions, and achieve higher muscle hypertrophy.

Additionally, adequate hydration is essential for improving the supply of nutrients to muscles and speeding up the healing process. Essential nutrients, including proteins, carbohydrates, and electrolytes, are transported to muscle cells through the medium of water, where they are used for the creation of energy, the repair of damaged tissue, and the synthesis of new muscle.

After exercise, staying properly hydrated helps flush out metabolic waste products like lactic acid, which lowers the chance of muscle stiffness and tiredness and speeds up recovery in between training sessions.

Apart from its immediate influence on physical performance, sufficient hydration promotes general health and wellness, which are essential components of women's bodybuilding. Maintaining appropriate cardiovascular function, controlling body temperature, and bolstering immunological function—all of which are linked to overall athletic performance and resilience—require proper hydration.

Furthermore, maintaining hydration can help women bodybuilders avoid typical problems like weariness, cramping in the muscles, and heat-related illnesses, making training more pleasurable and long-lasting.

Proper hydration affects performance, recuperation, and general health, making it essential for women to succeed in the bodybuilding industry. Women can improve their ability to perform well in training and competition, support nutrition delivery and recuperation, and maximize muscle function by making regular water consumption a priority.

For women who want to achieve their bodybuilding objectives while putting performance and wellbeing first, it is crucial to incorporate hydration measures into a thorough nutrition and training plan.

Electrolytes and Hydration Balance

With the help of this in-depth guide, we will examine the significance of electrolyte balance and the function it plays in maintaining optimal performance and general health for female bodybuilders.

Recognizing Hydration

Drinking water is only one aspect of being hydrated; another is keeping the body's delicate fluid and electrolyte balance intact in order to support vital physiological processes. Sufficient hydration is essential for controlling body temperature, lubricating joints, delivering nutrients, and eliminating metabolic waste products in the context of women's bodybuilding. Hydration should be prioritized as part of a comprehensive diet and training strategy because dehydration can result in lower performance, delayed recovery, and an increased risk of injury.

Electrolytes' Function:

Electrolytes are essential for maintaining proper hydration and good muscle function. These include sodium, potassium, calcium, magnesium, and chloride. Women lose electrolytes through sweat after vigorous exercise; these must be replaced to preserve electrolyte balance and avoid dehydration.

In instance, sodium aids in water retention and fluid balance, whereas potassium promotes nerve and muscle function. While chloride aids in maintaining the body's pH levels and fluid equilibrium, calcium, magnesium, and other elements are involved in the contraction and relaxation of muscles.

Hydration Strategies for Women in Bodybuilding:

Pre-Workout Hydration: To guarantee ideal fluid levels, begin hydrating well in advance of your exercise activity. Try to have 16–20 ounces of water two to three hours before working out, and another 8–10 ounces ten to twenty minutes before you begin.

Drink plenty of water throughout your workout to replenish any fluids lost through perspiration. When exercising, try to consume 7–10 ounces of water every 10–20 minutes, varying the amount according to your perspiration rate, level of effort, and the surroundings.

Post-Workout Hydration: Replace electrolytes and fluids lost during exercise by rehydrating as soon as possible. When exercising, try to drink 16–24 ounces of water for each pound of weight lost. You should also think about refueling with electrolyte-rich fluids or sports drinks, which contain potassium, sodium, and other essential electrolytes.

Keep an eye on your level of hydration. Look out for symptoms of dehydration, such as headaches, cramping in the muscles, dark urine, and dry mouth. To stay optimally hydrated throughout the day, monitor your fluid intake and modify your hydration plan as necessary.

Replace Electrolytes: To maintain hydration and restore electrolyte storage, include meals and drinks high in electrolytes in your diet. To guarantee proper electrolyte intake, include foods like bananas, oranges, yogurt, almonds, seeds, leafy greens, and sports drinks with added electrolytes.

Think About Individual Needs: Keep in mind that different people require different amounts of water based on their body weight, perspiration rate, level of exercise, climate, and other variables. Pay attention to your body's demands and preferences when adjusting your hydration plan.

Women bodybuilders can boost muscle recovery, improve general health and well-being, and maximize their performance by emphasizing hydration and electrolyte balance. To keep hydrated, energetic, and prepared to meet your fitness objectives, incorporate these hydration measures into your diet and exercise regimen. Remember, being hydrated is essential to your success as a female bodybuilder and is not just a part of your training program.

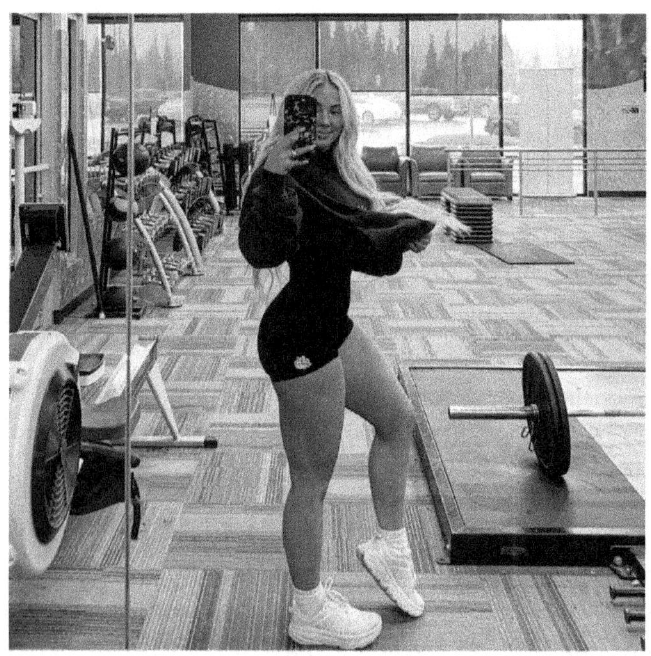

CHAPTER SEVEN

SUPPLEMENTS FOR WOMEN'S BODYBUILDING

Protein Supplements: Types and Usage

Achieving fitness objectives and improving outcomes require an understanding of the kinds and use of protein supplements. This thorough guide examines the different kinds of protein supplements, their uses, advantages, and things to keep in mind for female bodybuilders.

Importance of Protein in Women's Bodybuilding:

The building blocks of muscle tissue growth and repair are found in protein.

Consuming enough protein aids in the body's recovery from strenuous exercise.

Protein helps burn fat from the body while preserving lean muscular mass.

Types of Protein Supplements:

a. Whey Protein:

Obtained from milk and used in the production of cheese.

Quick absorption, which makes it perfect for recuperating after exercise.

Has all the necessary amino acids, with a high leucine content that is important for the synthesis of muscle protein.

Ideal for females who want to gain and keep lean muscular mass.

b. Casein Protein:

Similar to whey but more slowly absorbed and digested than milk.

Gives an extended release of amino acids, which is advantageous for muscle repair that takes place over night.

Might be taken in place of meals or before fasting times like bed.

c. Soy Protein:

Vegetable protein that is acceptable for vegans and vegetarians.

Includes every necessary amino acid.

May also lower cholesterol and promote heart health, among other health advantages.

Perfect for ladies with dietary restrictions or dairy allergy.

d. Pea Protein:

An additional plant-based choice that is acceptable for vegans and vegetarians.

Methionine content is reduced, but all necessary amino acids are present.

Suitable for people with dairy allergy or lactose intolerance, and easily digested.

May encourage sensations of fullness and support healthy weight management.

e. Hemp Protein:

Produced from the hemp plant's seeds.

Has a high content of omega-3 and omega-6 fatty acids and all the necessary amino acids.

May also improve heart health and reduce inflammation, among other health advantages.

Ideal for people who are allergic to soy or dairy products.

Choosing the Right Protein Supplement:

When choosing a protein supplement, take into account dietary constraints, personal preferences, and fitness objectives.

Carefully read ingredient labels to make sure the product satisfies personal preferences and demands.

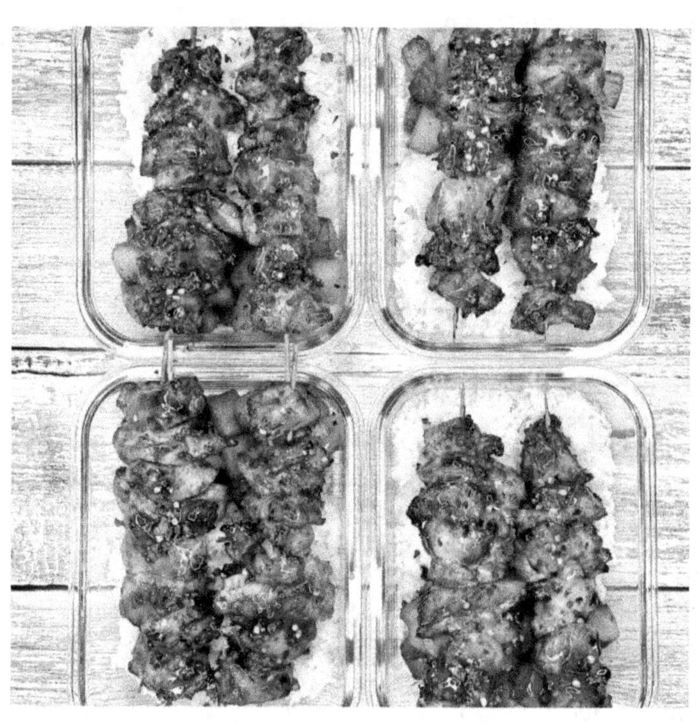

Try out a variety of protein supplement kinds to see which one is best for flavor, digestibility, and efficacy.

Post-Workout: Within 30 to 60 minutes following a workout, consuming a protein shake will aid start the process of muscle repair and recovery.

Meal Replacement: When entire food sources are unavailable or there are hectic days ahead, protein supplements might be a practical meal replacement.

Before Bed: To promote muscle regeneration during the night and stop muscle breakdown during fasting periods, casein protein is frequently advised before bed.

Protein Requirements: In order to maintain muscle growth and repair, female bodybuilders may have higher protein requirements than do inactive people.

Hormonal Factors: Women's varying hormone levels can affect how well proteins are metabolized and used, which highlights the significance of maintaining a steady protein intake during the menstrual cycle.

Individual Needs: Adjust protein consumption according to exercise levels, body composition, and personal fitness objectives.

Protein supplements are useful tools for female bodybuilders since they supply vital nutrients that aid in muscle growth, repair, and general performance. Women can improve their nutrition to efficiently reach their fitness objectives by knowing the many kinds of protein supplements, their advantages, and how to use them. A licensed dietitian or other healthcare professional can offer specific advice on how to incorporate protein supplements into a healthy diet and exercise routine.

Essential Vitamins and Mineral Supplements

These nutrients are essential for maintaining overall health, recuperation, and muscle growth. The essential vitamins and minerals listed below are ones that female bodybuilders should think about taking supplements of to make sure their nutritional demands are fully satisfied.

Calcium:

Supports the health of the muscles and bones.

It's particularly important for women to avoid osteoporosis.

Magnesium

Helps produce energy, relax muscles, and synthesise proteins.

Frequently exhausted during vigorous exercise.

Iron:

Vital for generating energy and transporting oxygen.

Women who have heavy menstrual cycles in particular might need to take supplements.

Zinc

Supports the manufacture of proteins, hormone control, and the immune system.

Excessive exertion may raise the excretion of zinc, requiring supplementation.

Vitamin D

vital for immune system health, bone density, and muscle function.

especially important for people who don't get much sun exposure.

B complex vitamin:

Contains the B vitamins—B6, B12, and folate—which are essential for the synthesis of red blood cells and the utilization of energy.

Promotes recuperation and general energy levels.

Women's bodybuilders need to include vital vitamins and minerals in their supplement routine to support their intense training, muscle growth, and general health. Women can enhance their bodybuilding journey by optimizing their performance, recuperation, and overall health by making sure they consume enough of these nutrients.

It is essential to speak with a medical expert or qualified dietitian to ascertain your unique supplement needs depending on your goals, food, and lifestyle.

CHAPTER EIGHT

BALANCING HORMONES THROUGH NUTRITION

These imbalances can cause a wide range of health problems, from weariness and mood swings to more serious illnesses like metabolic diseases and infertility. It is impossible to overestimate the importance of nutrition on hormonal health, even while lifestyle and heredity play major roles.

This thorough book seeks to examine the complex interplay between hormone balance and nutrition, offering insightful advice on how to best promote normal hormonal function through dietary choices.

Understanding Hormonal Health:

It's important to comprehend the intricate interactions between hormones in the body before exploring the influence of nutrition. Hormones are chemical messengers that are produced by the pancreas, thyroid, adrenal glands, and reproductive organs, among other glands.

Numerous body processes, such as metabolism, energy levels, mood, sleep patterns, and reproductive health, are regulated by these hormones. However, a number of things can upset the delicate balance of hormones, including stress, poor eating habits, lack of sleep, and exposure to pollutants in the environment. This can result in dysregulation and negative health repercussions.

Nutrition and Hormonal Balance:

By giving the body the vital nutrients required for hormone synthesis, metabolism, and signaling, nutrition plays a critical role in preserving hormonal balance. Dietary decisions play a critical role in hormone optimization since specific food ingredients have the potential to either support or undermine hormonal health.

Here's a closer look at how particular eating habits and foods affect hormone balance:

The macronutrients

Protein: Consuming enough protein is essential for the synthesis and control of hormones. Foods high in protein supply the amino acids needed to make hormones such as growth hormone, insulin, and thyroid hormones.

Fats: Good fats are essential for hormone production and cellular signaling. Examples of these fats include omega-3 fatty acids, which are present in walnuts, flaxseeds, and fatty fish. They help maintain the integrity of cell membranes, which promotes the activity of hormone receptors, and they are precursors to hormones like prostaglandins.

Carbs: Stable blood sugar levels and prolonged energy levels are supported by complex carbs found in whole grains, fruits, and vegetables. These blood sugar levels are essential for insulin regulation and hormonal balance in general.

Micronutrients:

Vitamins and Minerals: A number of components of hormonal health depend on nutrients such as vitamin D, vitamin B6, magnesium, zinc, and selenium. For instance, zinc and magnesium are important for thyroid and insulin sensitivity, while vitamin D aids in the synthesis of steroid hormones.

Phytonutrients: Plant-based substances that influence hormone activity and support hormonal balance include phytoestrogens, which are found in soy products, lignans in flaxseeds, and polyphenols in fruits and vegetables.

Gastrointestinal wellness

In the metabolism and communication of hormones, the gut microbiota is essential. A varied and healthy gut flora is supported by a diet high in fruits, vegetables, and whole grains. This, in turn, affects hormone balance and metabolism.

Foods That Support Hormones:

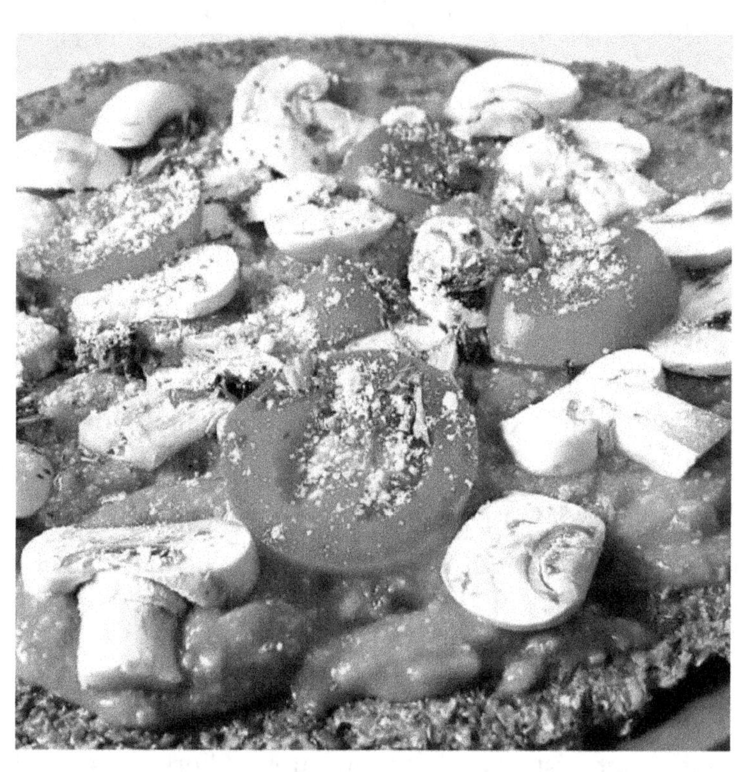

Compounds in some diets directly help hormonal balance. As examples, consider:

Broccoli, kale, and cauliflower are examples of cruciferous vegetables. They include sulfur compounds that aid in the liver's detoxification of excess hormones.

Berries and other fruits high in antioxidants fight oxidative stress and inflammation, which can throw off the balance of hormones.

Because of their probiotic content, fermented foods like yogurt, kefir, and sauerkraut improve hormonal balance and gut health.

Hydration:

Hormone balance and general health depend on enough hydration. Water helps the body eliminate metabolic waste products and facilitates the movement of hormones throughout the body, all of which contribute to the best possible functioning of hormones.

Steer Clear of Hormone Interruptors:

Hormonal equilibrium can be upset by certain dietary and environmental conditions. These include consuming large amounts of alcohol, consuming processed foods high in sugar and unhealthy fats, and being exposed to chemicals that alter hormones that are included in plastics, pesticides, and personal care items.

Incorporating Hormone-Balancing Nutrition into Your Lifestyle:

Hormone balance can be achieved and maintained through nutrition, but it takes a comprehensive strategy that includes careful food selection, lifestyle adjustments, and routine hormonal health monitoring. The following useful advice will help you include hormone-balancing foods into your daily routine:

Make a point of consuming full, nutrient-dense foods, such as whole grains, lean meats, healthy fats, and an assortment of fruits and vegetables.

Make eating organic and locally grown food a priority to reduce your exposure to pesticides and other dangerous substances.

Include foods high in phytonutrients and hormone-supporting elements in your diet, such as fermented foods, berries, and cruciferous vegetables.

Make sure you consume enough water throughout the day—at least 8 to 10 glasses—to stay hydrated.

Refined sweets, processed meals, and unhealthy fats should be avoided as they might upset hormone balance and cause inflammation.

Eat mindfully, observing your body's signals of hunger and fullness, and abstaining from emotional eating.

To maintain healthy cortisol levels and hormonal balance overall, manage stress with mindfulness exercises, regular exercise, enough sleep, and relaxation techniques.

See a medical practitioner or certified nutritionist for individualized advice and suggestions based on your particular hormonal profile and desired level of health.

Hormone balance through nutrition is a dynamic and complex process that includes establishing a lifestyle that promotes hormonal health, selecting nutrient-rich foods, and making educated dietary choices.

Through a comprehensive comprehension of the complex correlation between hormones and nutrition, as well as the application of pragmatic tactics to enhance food consumption, people can proactively strive for and sustain hormonal equilibrium, therefore advancing their general health and welfare.

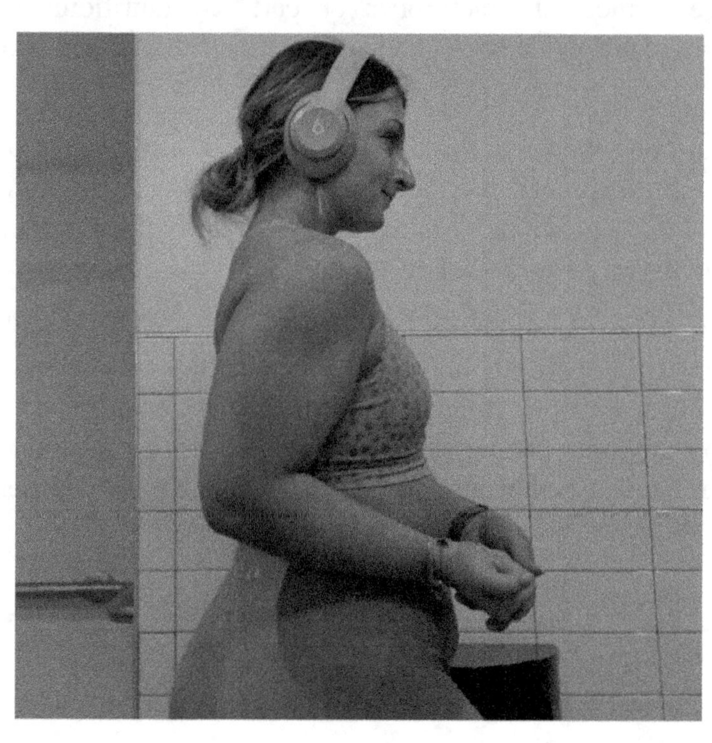

CHAPTER NINE

HEALTHY SNACKING AND EATING ON THE GO

Nutrient-Dense Snack Options

However, it is feasible to make nutrient-dense decisions that promote your general well-being with a little preparation and awareness. Providing a thorough understanding of nutrient-dense snacks that can nourish your body and satiate your appetites even while you're busy is the main goal of this book.

Recognizing Nutrient-Dense Snacks:

Snacks that are high in nutrients in comparison to their calorie level are considered nutrient-dense. These snacks are high in fiber, vitamins, minerals, and other vital nutrients that your body requires to operate at its best. Nutrient-dense snacks support your general health and keep you energized throughout the day, in contrast to empty-calorie foods like sweets or chips that have less nutritional value.

Comprehensive Nutrient-Dense Snack Options:

Fresh Fruits:

Fruits like apples, bananas, oranges, berries, and grapes are easy choices that need little preparation.

They provide you a rapid energy boost and encourage satiety because they are high in vitamins, antioxidants, and fiber.

Raw Vegetables:

Crunchy, low-calorie snacks like carrot sticks, celery, cucumber slices, and bell pepper strips are great options.

They are the best for sating hunger in between meals because they are high in fiber, vitamins, and minerals.

Nuts and Seeds:

Rich in nutrients, almonds, walnuts, pistachios, pumpkin seeds, and sunflower seeds are good sources of fiber, protein, and healthy fats.

When ingested in moderation, they support heart health and offer prolonged energy.

Greek Yogurt:

Greek yogurt is a delicious, high-protein snack that tastes great on its own or with nuts and fruits mixed in.

Because of its rich calcium, protein, and probiotic content, it supports gut and bone health.

Hummus and Whole Grain Crackers:

Chickpea hummus is a tasty dip that goes great with vegetable sticks or whole grain crackers.

It's a wonderful source of fiber, healthy fats, and plant-based protein that helps with digestion and fullness.

Cottage Cheese with Fruit:

A sweet and salty delicacy can be created by combining cottage cheese with dried or fresh fruits. Cottage cheese is a flexible snack.

It helps with muscle growth and repair because of its high protein, calcium, and B vitamin content.

Hard-Boiled Eggs:

Pliable and easy to carry, hard-boiled eggs are a great source of protein, vitamins, and minerals for snacks.

They are a great choice for hectic days because they contribute to satiety and offer sustained energy.

Tips for Healthy Snacking on the Go:

Make a plan and prepare nutrient-dense snacks ahead of time to help you resist the urge to go for harmful options.

Select snacks that provide you with a balanced diet and long-lasting energy by combining protein, fiber, and healthy fats.

To optimize nutritional advantages, use whole, minimally processed meals whenever possible.

Water is a good way to stay hydrated throughout the day because often people confuse thirst with appetite.

In order to eat mindfully—savoring every bite and avoiding distractions—pay attention to your body's hunger cues.

It doesn't have to be difficult to have healthful snacks while on the run. Nutrient-dense foods like whole grains, fresh produce, nuts, yogurt, and fruits will fuel your body and promote general health and wellbeing. You may have tasty and filling snacks that keep you nourished and energized throughout your busy day with a little preparation and attentive eating.

Smart Choices for Eating Out

Investigating Restaurant Options:

- Talk about how it's critical to look up healthier options on restaurant menus ahead of time.

- Provide methods, like utilizing applications or internet resources, for locating eateries that serve wholesome options.

Comprehending Menu Terminology:

- Interpret frequently used terms and phrases from menus that pertain to nutrition and health (e.g., "grilled" versus "fried," "steamed" versus "sautéed").

- Provide assistance in perusing menus to find items that fit your goals and dietary restrictions.

Tailor Your Order:

– Encourage readers to take charge of their meals and make them healthier by asking for sauces or dressings on the side, choosing whole-grain choices, or changing ingredients.

Mindful Eating Practices:

- Examine the idea of mindful eating and how it might help you eat healthily and more thoroughly.

- Give advice on how to be attentive when eating out, such as slowing down, enjoying every bite, and observing your body's signals of hunger and fullness.

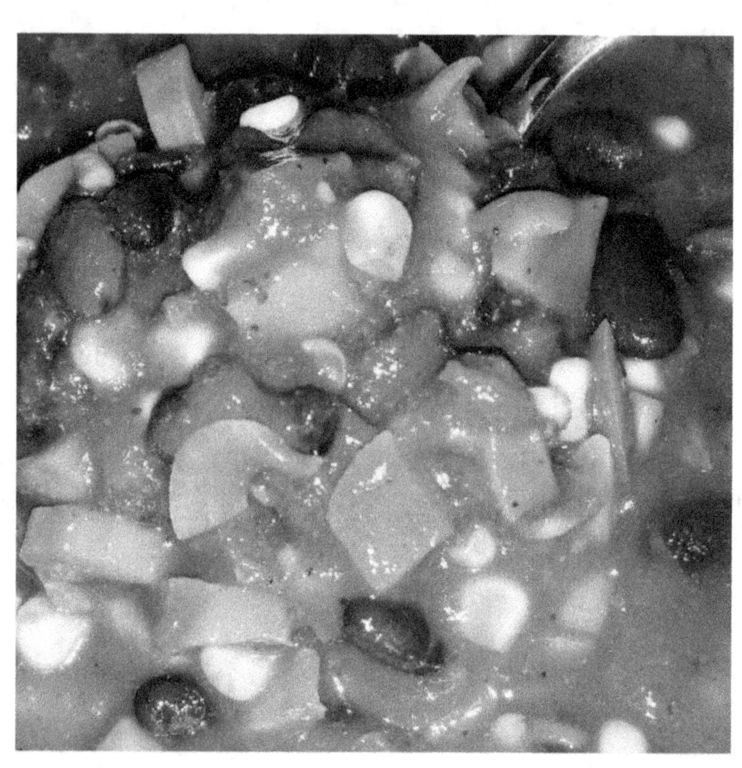

CHAPTER TEN

MONITORING PROGRESS AND ADJUSTING NUTRITION PLANS

There's more to starting a bodybuilding adventure than merely lifting weights and sticking to a cookie cutter diet. For female bodybuilders, tracking their development and making necessary dietary adjustments are essential to getting the best results. We'll explore the significance of monitoring and evaluating fitness objectives in this in-depth guide, as well as how to adjust food regimens for ongoing progress that are especially catered to female bodybuilders.

Understanding Fitness Goals:

Clearly Define Your Goals: Prior to beginning any fitness program, you should set SMART (specific, measurable, achievable, relevant, and time-bound) objectives. These objectives can be to increase muscular mass, decrease body fat, build strength, or get ready for a competition.

Evaluate Initial Metrics: Assess your current strength, weight, body composition, and eating patterns first. This gives you a starting point from which to monitor your development and make wise decisions as you go.

Include Variability: For best results, female bodybuilders should concentrate on a well-rounded fitness regimen that includes strength training, cardio, flexibility training, and enough rest.

Tracking Development:

Track Body Composition: To keep an eye on changes over time, measure your total weight, muscular mass, and body fat % on a regular basis. Skinfold calipers, bioelectrical impedance analysis (BIA), and DEXA scans are a few techniques that can be used for this.

Maintain a Workout Log: Keep track of the exercises, sets, repetitions, and weights used during your workouts. Monitoring development enables changes in response to performance gains or plateaus.

Evaluate Performance and Strength: Monitor strength gains by timing your workouts or testing your one-rep maximum (1RM) on a regular basis to gauge your endurance. Performance improvement is a sign of a well-executed training and diet program.

Modifying Dietary Routines:

Macronutrients and Calorie Intake: Determine your daily energy requirements depending on your exercise level and goals. Make sure you are getting enough of the macronutrients (protein, carbs, and fats) to help with energy levels, muscle building, and recuperation.

Protein Requirements: In order to assist muscle growth and repair, bodybuilding women usually need to consume more protein. For each kilogram of body weight, aim for 1.2–2.2 grams of protein per day, split equally between meals.

Carbohydrate Timing: To maximize training sessions and restore glycogen stores, carefully schedule your intake of carbohydrates around physical activity. For long-lasting energy, prioritize complex carbs and limit your sugar intake.

Healthy Fats: To promote hormone production, joint health, and general well-being, include sources of healthy fats like avocados, nuts, seeds, and fatty fish in your diet.

Micronutrient Balance: Make sure you're getting a wide range of vitamins and minerals from whole grains, fruits, vegetables, and, if necessary, supplements. Keep an eye out for micronutrients like calcium, magnesium, and potassium that are essential for proper muscular function.

Constant Enhancement:

Regular Assessments: To pinpoint areas for progress, periodically reevaluate your body composition, performance metrics, and fitness goals.

Progressive Overload: To promote muscular growth and inhibit adaptation, gradually increase the volume, resistance, or intensity of your workouts. This will continuously test your body.

Pay Attention to Comments: Observe the body's reaction to dietary and workout modifications. Plan modifications based on input to maximize outcomes and guard against injury or exhaustion.

Consult a Professional: For individualized advice and assistance, think about speaking with a licensed nutritionist, dietitian, or personal trainer with experience in women's bodybuilding.

Tracking results and modifying diet regimens are essential elements of a successful female bodybuilding journey. Women can prioritize their health and well-being while achieving their desired body by setting clear goals, monitoring their progress, and making educated modifications.

To get lasting effects, keep in mind that patience and consistency are crucial, and that you must pay attention to your body's signals at every stage of the process.

CONCLUSION

Embracing a disciplined, committed, and self-care-focused lifestyle is just as important as changing one's physical appearance when following a bodybuilding diet designed especially for women. We have covered the essential concepts of tracking advancement and modifying diet regimens in this guide to help women effectively reach their bodybuilding objectives.

Women can change their lives by learning how to create specific goals for their fitness, monitor their progress using different metrics, and make educated nutritional changes in order to increase their strength, improve the definition of their muscles, and improve their general health.

It is important for women to keep in mind that the mental toughness they develop along the route is just as important to success as any physical changes they make while navigating the complexities of the bodybuilding path. When people work to achieve their goals, consistency, tolerance, and flexibility are essential.

Sustainable growth in the pursuit of continual improvement necessitates listening to one's body, seeking professional help when necessary, and embracing a holistic approach to wellness.

In the end, this book is a thorough manual and friend for female bodybuilders, encouraging them to take control of their health, push their boundaries, and recognize their inner strength. May this trip be a life-changing experience that

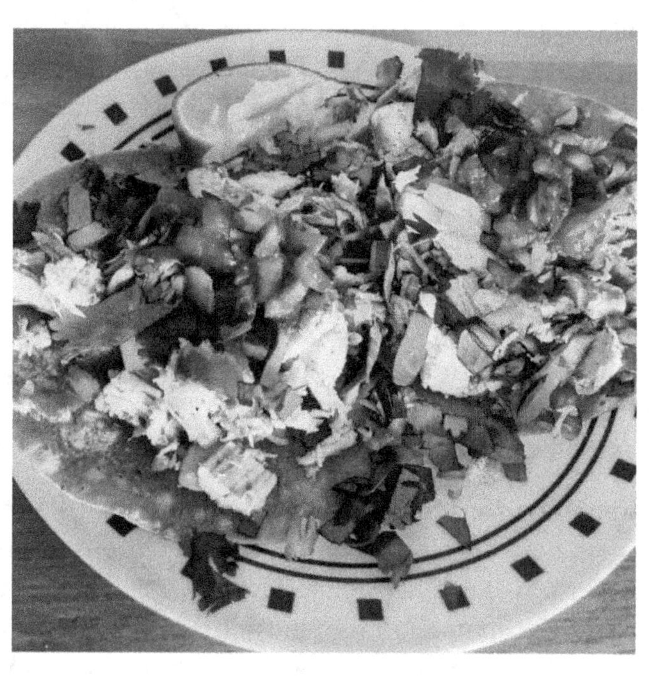

promotes development, resiliency, and self-discovery rather than being a means to an end.

Let's honor the incredible journey that female bodybuilders have taken and all of the opportunities that lie ahead for those that aspire to be the best.

HAPPY READING!!!